Sleep Peacefully

Your Guide to Sleeping Peacefully in Mind, Body, and Spirit

MARK BALDWIN, LPC-MHSP

ACKNOWLEDGEMENTS

John 16:33 says "In this world you will have trouble. But take heart I have overcome the world." Without God nothing I have done would be possible or beneficial. My wife and three kids have literally stood by my side in ways that I cannot explain. For that I am truly grateful! I love you all.

Contents

CHAPTER 1: INTRODUCTION

It's about 1am and as he rolls over and wakes up he sees a bluish light shining on the ceiling of the bedroom. At first he's not sure what it is and then it hits him, it's the glow of his wife's cell phone. She can't sleep and she's killing time by playing on her phone. Now every time he sees that glowing lights he jokes that the aliens are invading again. Unfortunately, difficulty sleeping is an all too common problem. Part of the issue is today's culture, which is

Sleep Needed By Age Group

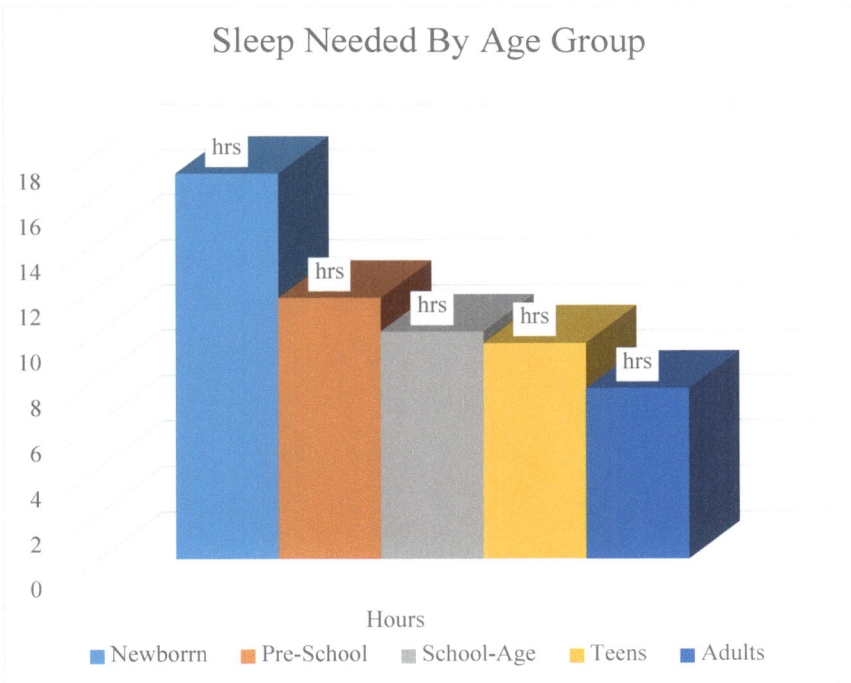

filled distractions and overall busyness. As a matter of fact, the problem is so serious that the CDC has an entire department dedicated to sleep problems. This is a major health issue – mentally, physically, and spiritually! "About 70 million Americans suffer from chronic sleep problems."[i] Consistent lack of sleep has been linked to numerous health issues, both physical and mental, including increases in risky behaviors, problems with weight gain, heart disease, depression, anxiety, decreased reaction time leading to accidents, and more!

Far too often people only take into consideration one area of their life as it relates to sleep – the physical side, or body. As a result many people consider medication as the only solution. At LifeWorks Resources, we want to encourage a holistic approach involving mind, body, and spirit. Therefore, let's take a look at the three areas by first recognizing the problems that lack of sleep causes our mind, body, and spirit, and then we will explore solutions for all three areas. As always, be sure to discuss these areas with your physician, counselor, and pastor to make sure that your sleep plan fits in to your overall wellness plan.

Your Mind and Sleep – The Problem:

When we talk about the mind, we are referring to both your thoughts and your emotions. We'll leave the physical attributes of your brain in the concept of your physical body, which will be covered later. Why do we say that the mind includes emotions? There are two main reasons. First, many counselors believe that the emotions are controlled by thoughts. For example, if you are driving and get cut off by another driver, your thoughts actually drive your emotional response. If you immediately think of the other driver as an "idiot" and "dangerous" then anger may be your emotional response. Second, we do know that our emotions are a core function and at times may cause us to think things based on our emotions. Confused yet? Remember that the mind is one of the most complex parts of people. SO which comes first...thoughts or emotions. The truth is that no one knows for sure and most of what is in the research is all theories. Here is what you need to know: your mind and emotions are connected and they have a major impact on your sleep. Also, your lack of sleep and/or poor quality sleep impacts your mind!

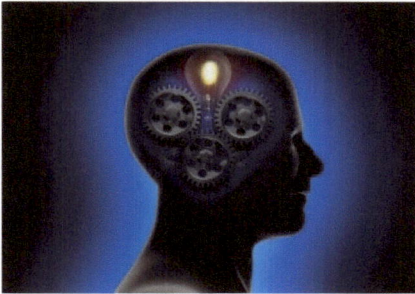

One research study concluded the following: "Disturbed sleep is an important predictor of fatigue, apparently stronger than previously well-established predictors such as work load, female gender, lack of exercise, etc."[ii] This research is referring to a person's mental tiredness as a result of poor or lack of sleep. Think about what this means about your life. If you are lacking sleep or not sleeping well, then your daily performance will suffer. If you work in an office setting, then no doubt you have notices yourself or others nodding off or daydreaming at times during the day. Or maybe it's just a slower pace so as to combat the mental tiredness that has taken over. Not only that, according to the above research, mental tiredness is more closely related to sleep problems than many other factors that have been looked at regarding tiredness. This mental fatigue means that you may struggle at work and in your relationships. When people are tired they do not think as clearly, and they do not deal with problems and stress well. When one person in a relationship is tired due to a lack of sleep, he or she may react poorly and impatiently with people they are closest to! It is amazing the number of people who come to counseling that struggle with sleep problems. The stress has impacted so many areas of their life that they seek counseling not for sleep but for the negative impact the stress is having on themselves and their relationships. Questions about sleep are now a part of all medical and counseling intake questionnaires because it's broad implications on overall well-being.

Another research article reported that "...sleep deprivation induces specific risks for automatic, skill-based behavior that are not present in consciously controlled performance."[iii] What this means is that a person's ability to learn mental sequencing tasks – like an ordered list – is greatly reduced when people are tired due to a lack of sleep or poor quality sleep. Again, poor sleep leads to problems and struggles in a person's thinking. When someone struggles with sleep, they may experience problems remembering things in the correct order. Unfortunately, some may wrongly think that they are losing their memory or think they are stupid because of the struggles to learn sequences when actually the problem is poor quality sleep or a lack of sleep.

Not only do sleep difficulties cause problems with your mind, but your mind can cause problems with your sleep. Stress, anxiety, and worry can cause problems falling asleep, staying asleep - or both – and cause you to wake up earlier than you intended. These problems that may be making sleep more difficult for you are all related to your mind, including your emotions. The problem then is not only sleep but also what is going on mentally and emotionally throughout the day and especially what you may be thinking and feeling at bedtime. If you are overly stressed out at work or in your relationships then this stress will carry well beyond the situations throughout the day and cause problems with your ability to sleep and/or cause poor quality sleep.

Your Body and Sleep – The Problem:

When we talk about the body and its relationship to your sleep we are referring to physical body, food intake, and the environment around us that impacts a person's physical ability to sleep. This is similar to the way a medical doctor would look at the body, and we also include some other areas in this as well. Also, we will not talk about medications since we recommend that you discuss that and your overall plan with your physician.

We mentioned earlier that a lack of sleep or poor quality sleep can have an impact on your physical health, but here are some additional important points. One research study concluded that "These data suggest that lack of sleep in hypertensive patients may increase sympathetic nervous activity during the night and the following morning, leading to increased blood pressure and heart rate. "[iv] So if you already have high blood pressure, it may actually get worse overnight if you are not getting enough sleep or you are not getting peaceful sleep. This is dangerous and you need to be aware of these issues. The good news is that if you can improve

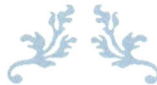

The Centers for Disease Control and Prevention notes that the lack of sleep in the U.S. is at epidemic levels!

your sleep then you may be able to avoid this problem. The Centers for Disease Control and Prevention (CDC) says this about your health and sleep problems: "Persons experiencing sleep insufficiency are also more likely to suffer from chronic diseases such as hypertension, diabetes, depression, and obesity, as well as from cancer, increased mortality, and reduced quality of life and productivity."[v] These are not minor health issues and the CDC notes that this is an epidemic!

This graphic helps to show the effects of sleep deprivation on the body. However, note that this is not just talking about some experiment where they keep people awake for days and see what happens. This can happen as a result of consistent lack of sleep or difficulty falling asleep or staying asleep.

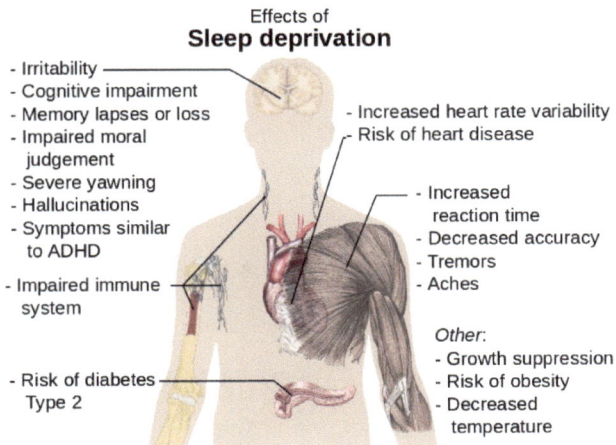

Effects of
Sleep deprivation

- Irritability
- Cognitive impairment
- Memory lapses or loss
- Impaired moral judgement
- Severe yawning
- Hallucinations
- Symptoms similar to ADHD

- Impaired immune system

- Risk of diabetes Type 2

- Increased heart rate variability
- Risk of heart disease

- Increased reaction time
- Decreased accuracy
- Tremors
- Aches

Other:
- Growth suppression
- Risk of obesity
- Decreased temperature

Your Spirit and Sleep – The Problem:

Far too often people do not consider their spiritual health when thinking about their inability to sleep well or lack of sleep. Sometimes people consider unhealthy spirituality or an unsettled spirit in the same category as their mind and emotions. Usually putting the health of one's spirit in the wrong category is done unintentionally. This can become a barrier to correcting difficulty with sleep or poor quality sleep. Dr Rubin Naiman believes, "...conventional medical approaches have fallen short by over emphasizing objective views of sleep while virtually ignoring the personal spiritual experience of the sleeper."[vi] Some have gone as far as to say that sleep is a spiritual act. These people make this connection because of the Biblical references to God speaking to His people through dreams while they sleep. If one thinks of their spirituality as a personal relationship with God, it makes sense that if there is strife in our heart with or toward God then we may struggle to sleep peacefully. Similarly, if someone is struggling with idols (putting something else as more important than God), then the relationship struggles and your spirit may be unsettled. For example, a person can become overly focused on themselves. This self-centeredness is idolatry and can often lead to poor sleep or a lack of sleep. This is likely a major struggle in today's culture due to increased information and technology and the ability to meet many of our wants nearly instantaneously. This makes it very easy for people to fall into the trap of selfishness.

Summary and Keys to Remember:

As you can see, sleep issues are a major problem that we need to be aware of and take the steps necessary to return balance to this part of our lives – to be able to sleep peacefully! This balance needs to include more than just taking a pill at night and hoping for the best. There are additional, healthy, holistic approaches that can be beneficial. Certainly talk with your doctor and decide what is best for your particular, situation but this resource can help you learn to sleep peacefully by giving you some ideas and research to help you solve this issue.

As you think about the problems stated above and look forward to the solutions to follow, try not to get discouraged. Remember that this is a solvable problem. Although it may take some time to figure out exactly what works for you, it will help you become a healthier and ultimately happier you. Also, remember

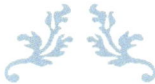

Remember that this is a solvable problem and although it may take some time to figure out exactly what works for you, it will help you become a healthier and happier you!

that you are not alone! Nearly 70 million Americans have this same problem!

As you begin to look at the solutions, do not try to change everything at once. Instead make small changes and be patient with the results. You will want to give the things you try time to work and your mind, body, and spirit time to change the habits you have already created. Remember that research suggests that it takes approximately one month to begin to create new habits. Give yourself enough time to try different approaches and then begin to change the habits to create a consistent lifestyle that promotes peaceful sleep. Change takes time, and there is not an immediate, quick fix. If there was, there would be no need for this resource and all the research that has been done to solve America's sleep problem!

Chapter 2: Your Mind and Peaceful Sleep

In this chapter we will begin exploring practical solutions to help you learn to fall asleep and stay asleep. Remember that practical does not necessarily mean easy. Depending on what your particular struggles are, some of the suggestions may not apply to you. Give them a try and figure out what works best for you. Also, remember that it takes about a month to create new habits so give yourself time. By keeping these things in mind, you will take away some of the pressure on yourself and help lower your stress about not sleeping. So let's get started!

1. Manage Your Thoughts

    Does your mind start to race through a myriad of thoughts as soon as you lay down and try to relax? For many this is due to two primary issues. First, you may not be managing your worry, stress, and anxiety throughout each day. As a result, your mind starts to process this information as soon as you have some "down time". Unfortunately in today's culture with the stress and the busy-ness that you face, you may not be taking enough time to process the day's events before you go to bed.

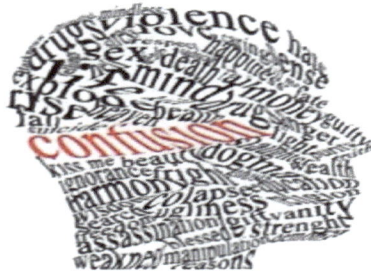

Second, you may have a tendency toward creativity when other distractions are gone and it is time to sleep. This is a tough one to deal with, because you do not want to lose the creative process and the helpful things your mind is inventing. Yet it is also an inconvenient and unhealthy process if it interferes with your sleep. Also, in the long run it will hurt your creative process because of the consequences of a lack of sleep or poor sleep. Here are some suggestions for you to try:

a. Know whether you are an internal or external processor.

In other words, some people process their thoughts without having to say things out loud or write them down. These people are internal processors and can work out a conversation entirely in their head. Others need to be able to say what they are thinking out loud to help them process their thoughts. Either way is fine, but it is helpful to know which one you are, as this will change which steps you want to try and how to go about it.

b. Try to get out of your head by taking your thoughts captive.

We cannot always control the thoughts that enter our mind initially, but we can decide what to do with those thoughts. By taking the thought captive, you then decide what to do with it. For example, you can throw it out as not worthy of any consideration, write it down to come back to later, decide that it's a negative thought and rethink it to make it positive, or you can choose to think about something that helps you relax. In all likelihood you will do some of each of these depending on the thought. Also, if you do decide to write the thought down, guard against going into detail about it by just making enough of a note that you can come back to it later. This is especially true if you are in a creative brainstorming session and do not want to lose the great ideas.

2. Think About Relaxing Not About Sleeping

You may be making the all too common mistake of thinking about sleeping. This just makes it more obvious that you are having trouble sleeping and becomes a distraction. It also raises your anxiety at the worst possible time. Try to think of things that will help you relax rather than focusing on the actual task at hand. One way to do that is through some simple meditation techniques covered a little later. Also, you can try to completely clear your mind, but this takes a lot of practice for some people and can be nearly impossible for others.

3. Remove Distractions

When life was simpler, people fell asleep because there was

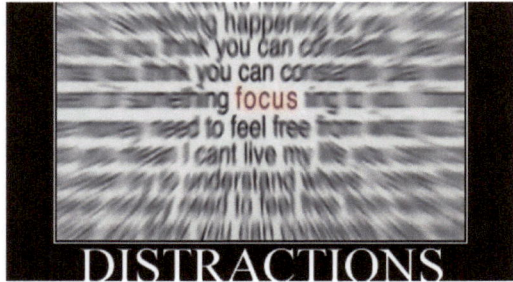

nothing to do once the lights went out. However, today we are bombarded with things to do other than sleep. It is amazing the number of people that have TVs in their bedroom. If you do, turn it off and resist the urge to turn it on at bedtime. This creates a distraction that your mind does not need, as you will be overwhelmed with information being shot at you without you even realizing it. Also, with the invention of cell phones and tablets, people are now surfing the internet, texting, and more while lying in bed. Again, these become mental distractions that do little to help you relax and fall asleep. If you must do some activity because you can't sleep – leave the bed – stay in low light and do something that requires little mental effort – a mental distraction until you get tired.

4. Mood Disorders and Sleep

According to the Division of Sleep Medicine at Harvard Medical School,

"Chronic insomnia may increase the risk of developing a mood disorder, such as anxiety or depression." **AND**

"Poor sleep and feelings of depression or anxiety can be helped through a variety of treatments, starting with improved sleep habits..."[vii]

This complicates things, because both seem to impact each other. So what's the solution? First, make sure to discuss this with your physician and/or counselor so that they can help you determine how these steps fit into your overall plan. As for practical steps:

a. Awareness is powerful. Take note of how your mood impacts your sleep and vice versa. Make a journal or chart to help with this.

b. Get the proper help for any mood problems you may be having. Many of the things listed in this booklet will help as well.

c. Do not try to solve one without taking care of the other. They each impact the other, so deal with both of them appropriately and at the same time.

5. Meditation

Meditation can be a powerful tool to help you sleep by relaxing your mind. One of the simplest methods of this called one word meditation. Simply put you will pick a word either with a positive meaning – such as "relax" – or meaningless word – such as "one". Focus on your breathing and repeat the word. Vary the intervals at which you repeat the word to make it most useful for yourself. If your mind begins to wander then increase the frequency of the word. You can also try different words each time to see if that makes any difference for your specific situation. Also, there are meditation CDs and mp3 audio available that can help you with relaxation and meditation. As a matter of fact, we have one being developed right now! Not only will meditation help relax your mind so you can sleep, but it will also help to relax your body.

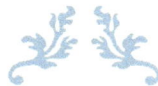

"The growth of the internet, 24-hour television channels and mobile phones means that we now receive five times as much information every day as we did in 1986." – The Deccan Herald

Chapter 3: Your Body and Peaceful Sleep

By now you know the negative impact of poor sleep on your body. In this chapter we will look at ways that you can change your body and environment to help you sleep. Think of the environmental aspect as a way of helping your body to relax. It sets the stage so to speak for the way that our body responds. Never forget that we are impacted mentally, emotionally, and spiritually by our surroundings. We will also include some foods that you can include in your diet to help you sleep better as well.

1. Make Sure You Have a Good Mattress

    People have said that a mattress is good for 10 years. However, according to 2008 Better Sleep Month (BSM) national survey, sponsored by the Better Sleep Council (BSC) people that reported sleeping well were more likely to be sleeping on a mattress less than four years old.[viii] A good mattress will help you be able to relax and help you to stay asleep.

2. Exercise

    Exercise helps so many things in our body such as weight, energy, and overall healthy. However

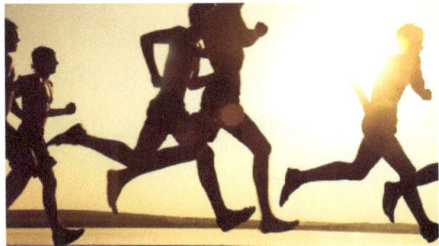

people often overlook its importance to your sleep. Exercise will improve your ability to fall asleep, and it will also improve the quality of your sleep. The only thing to be cautious of is to not exercise to close to bedtime as this can cause your body to be over energized and the release of endorphins in your brain may make falling asleep more difficult. If you are not a morning person and must exercise in the afternoon or after work, try to do it earlier rather than waiting until right before bedtime.

3. Light

Increase light exposure, specifically sunlight, throughout the day. Sunlight helps our biological clock and can also provide nutrients to our body. Protect yourself from sunburn but being in the sunlight helps your body in many ways. You may be spending too much time in dark areas or in artificial light – such as an office or a home that is not well lit. Although artificial light is better than low light throughout the day, it's no substitute for sunlight. Also, do just the opposite as it gets closer to bedtime – be in low light.

4. Routine

In today's world this can be very difficult for some people. Do not underestimate the importance of developing your own bedtime routine, including what time you will go to bed and what time you will wake up. Use the chart in chapter one to make sure your routine includes enough actual sleep time. A good routine will help your body adjust from the day's activities and stressors and provide you with time to wind down.

5. Comfort

Make sure that your bedroom is a place of peace and comfort. Besides your mattress and developing a good bedtime routine, pay attention to the overall ambiance or comfortability of your bedroom. Is it cluttered? Does it stress you out to lay in bed and look around? Do you feel relaxed in the environment where you're sleeping? Make sure your bedroom is a low light environment, and remember that cell phones, tablets, and computers destroy this environment. Also, make sure the temperature in your bedroom is comfortable. Pay attention to whether you get hot or cold when you sleep and make adjustments accordingly. Also, think about the smells in your bedroom. For some, candles or certain scents can help your body relax and yet others may struggle with allergies. Explore some of these suggestions to create the right environment for sleep.

Make sure that your bedroom is a place of peace!

6. Use Your Bed For Sleeping Only

    Earlier we talked about removing distractions to help your mind relax. This is closely related and seems to becoming more of a problem in today's technologically connected society. Try hard not to use your bed for reading or other wake time activities as it trains your body that the bed is for awake times. If you have ever heard of muscle memory this is the same concept. In muscle memory athletes use the same motion over and over to help their body learn what to do and eventually it becomes natural. The same is true when we use our bed for wake time activities. Instead, if you must do something at night, use low light in a place other than the bedroom. Also remember not to over stimulate during this time as it will interfere with peaceful sleep.

7. To Nap or Not to Nap

    Taking a nap can be a good thing but like so many good things in life, it is really about moderation and balance. There is no hard evidence that either option is better, but if you do choose to take a nap be cautious about it. Here are two easy things to remember when it comes to napping. First limit it to 20-30 minutes. Any longer, and it will interfere with your ability to sleep peacefully that night. You must be disciplined about this and not hit snooze on your alarm. Second, do not take a nap later in the day. It will confuse your body and disrupt a good night's sleep.

8. Eat Right

Just like exercise, eating well has many beneficial aspects. One of those is the impact it can have on your sleep. Therefore the first thing to remember is that an overall healthy diet will have a positive impact on your ability to fall asleep and the quality of that sleep. Also, there are some specific foods which you can add or remove from your diet to help as well.

   a. You may have heard of melatonin. It is a chemical in your brain that helps regulate your biological clock and it is also important to note that it has a tendency to decrease as you age. You can buy melatonin over-the-counter as a supplement. However, there are also foods that can help replenish melatonin in your body as well:

      i. Foods that contain B6 help your body produce melatonin. For example, fish is a good source of B6. So are bananas. Also, many fortified cereals contain B6 and can be a healthy way to start your day.

   b. Jasmine rice may increase tryptophan in your body. Tryptophan is what makes you want to sleep after eating turkey. However, Jasmine rice is probably a healthier alternative than eating turkey every evening.

c.   Research suggests that a lack of calcium may cause sleep problems. Make sure that you are getting enough calcium in your diet. One example is to eat yogurt, as it is a good source of calcium.

d.   Whole grains increase magnesium which may help with staying asleep. This may be a good solution for you if you struggle to stay asleep throughout the night.

e.   Lower your caffeine intake. For some the impact of caffeine on their body is obvious, while others may not realize its impact on the body. It is a stimulant and can make it difficult for you to fall asleep and stay asleep. If nothing else, make sure you do not have caffeine later in the day.

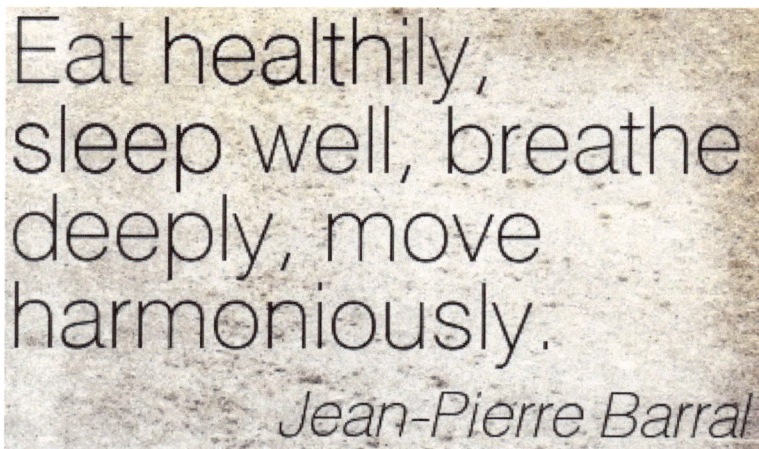

Eat healthily, sleep well, breathe deeply, move harmoniously.

Jean-Pierre Barral

f. Valerian root is an herb believed to act as a sedative for your body. This may be particularly useful if you struggle to fall asleep or it takes you a long time to get to sleep.

g. Finally, although it's not recommended that you eat a meal too close to bedtime, a healthy bedtime snack can help curb hunger while you sleep. Since hunger tends to wake you up at night, when a healthy snack is done wisely it can be beneficial.

Chapter 4: Your Spirit and Peaceful Sleep

We've reviewed how your mind and body can help you sleep, but one area often overlooked in the holistic approaches that currently exist is how what is going on spiritually may impact sleep. We're not here to question and probe into areas where you may be experiencing guilt or shame that is keeping you awake, but rather we want to explore positive ways to that your spiritual health can help you sleep peacefully. Of course, if you are struggling with guilt and/or shame please talk to your doctor, counselor, or pastor to help with that area of life. Often these are the areas that we suppress throughout the day, and then our spirit becomes uneasy when we lay our head on the pillow at night. Then suddenly, though exhausted, we can't sleep. Here are some verses to consider:

1. Psalm 4:8 – "In peace I will both lie down and sleep; for you alone, O LORD, make me dwell in safety."

   In a world full of turmoil, it is comforting to be reminded that God provides your safety. He is the one who ultimately provides peaceful sleep.

2. Proverbs 3:21-24 – "My son, do not lose sight of these- keep sound wisdom and discretion, and they will be life for your soul and adornment for your neck. Then you will walk on your way securely, and your foot will not stumble. If you lie

down, you will not be afraid; when you lie down, your sleep will be sweet.

Do you want sweet sleep? This verse points out that you must not lose sight of sound wisdom which is found in

God is the provider of peaceful sleep!

God and His word. His wisdom will help your soul and provide you with peaceful sleep.

3. Ecclesiastes 5:12a – "Sweet is the sleep of a laborer…"

   What a simple reminder that work is good for us. Take your work related stressors and be thankful for the job that you have and the opportunity to be a positive influence on those around you.

4. Jeremiah 31:25-26 – "For I will satisfy the weary soul, and every languishing soul I will replenish. At this I awoke and looked, and my sleep was pleasant to me."

   Do you feel weary and tired? Remember that He satisfies the soul and provides replenishing. "Replenish" would be a great word to meditate on with the one word meditation discussed earlier. The word languish can also refer to being stuck in a situation. Remember that He can replenish and work in every situation.

5. Exodus 33:14 – "And he said, 'My presence will go with you, and I will give you rest.'"

   Not only does He provide the peace that you need but He also says that He will go with you. Whether it's fear or worries or anxieties, or whatever may be causing you difficulty in sleep, He goes with you!

6. Joshua 1:13 – "Remember the word that Moses the servant of the LORD commanded you, saying, 'The LORD your God is providing you a place of rest and will give you this land.'"

   God is the provider. Too often we think of this in terms of money but this verse reminds us that He provides our rest. He also provides the strength you need to persevere and to be able to overcome the mental and physical battles that may be interfering with your sleep.

7. Psalm 116:7 – "Return, O my soul, to your rest; for the LORD has dealt bountifully with you."

   The Psalms are beautiful because you hear the cries to God for help and cries praising Him. This is both a cry for the soul to be returned to rest and thanks God that He has provided blessings. When we can be thankful even when we are crying out for help, we honor God.

8. Isaiah 57:1b-2 – "For the righteous man is taken away from calamity; he enters into peace; they rest in their beds who walk in their uprightness."

   To live righteously means that we are living according to God's ways. This does not mean you will be perfect, but rather that you try to please Him and acknowledge when you make a mistake. This way of living is what allows you to sleep peacefully. It is really about having the proper perspective.

9. Matthew 11:28-29 – "Come to me, all who labor and are heavy laden, and I will give you rest."

   Where do you turn when you are stressed out and exhausted? The answer to that question may well solve your sleep problems! This verse reminds you to go to Him. He has all the answers and wants you to come to Him and find rest in Him.

10. Psalm 37:11 – "But the meek shall inherit the land and delight themselves in abundant peace."

   Peaceful sleep starts with a peace in the spirit. This can be found by being gentle in spirit. Do not be a person who start trouble and strife. Be the person who is gentle in spirit and not only will you have peace but you will have more peace than you know what to do with!

ABOUT THE AUTHOR

Mark Baldwin is a Licensed Professional Counselor Mental Health Service Provider in Tennessee. He has worked in residential treatment for teens and private practice counseling. He now owns LifeWorks Resources which provides counseling and resources from a Biblical prospective. He earned a Bachelor degree in Psychology at the University of Minnesota – Duluth, a Master of Science degree in Counseling from Freed-Hardeman University, and an Ed.D. (ABD) in Counseling from the University of Memphis. Mark resides in Jackson Tennessee with his wife and three children, where they are actively involved at Northbrook Church.

LifeWorks Resources
www.lifeworksresources.com

END NOTES:

[i] Centers for Disease Control and Prevention. http://www.cdc.gov/sleep/about_us.htm (Retrieved 5/27/2014)

[ii] T. Åkerstedt, A. Knutsson, P. Westerholm, T. Theorell, L. Alfredsson, Göran Kecklund, Mental fatigue, work and sleep, Journal of Psychosomatic Research, Volume 57, Issue 5, November 2004, Pages 427-433, ISSN 0022-3999, http://dx.doi.org/10.1016/j.jpsychores.2003.12.001.

[iii] Effects of sleep loss, time of day, and extended mental work on implicit and explicit learning of sequences. Heuer, Herbert; Spijkers, Will; Kiesswetter, Ernst; Schmidtke, Volker. Journal of Experimental Psychology: Applied, Vol 4(2), Jun 1998, 139-162.

[iv] Effects of insufficient sleep on blood pressure in hypertensive patients: A 24-h study American Journal of Hypertension (1999) 12 (1): 63-68

[v] Centers for Disease Control and Prevention. Insufficient Sleep Is a Public Health Epidemic. http://www.cdc.gov/features/dssleep/

[vi] Sleep Review. New Book Integrates Spirituality Into Sleep. http://www.sleepreviewmag.com/2014/05/book-spirituality-sleep/

[vii] Mood and Sleep. Division of Sleep Medicine at Harvard Medical School. http://healthysleep.med.harvard.edu/need-sleep/whats-in-it-for-you/mood

[viii] Better Sleep Month national survey, sponsored by the Better Sleep Council. 2008. http://bettersleep.org/better-sleep/healthy-sleep/physical-performance-sleep/

www.ingramcontent.com/pod-product-compliance
Lightning Source LLC
Chambersburg PA
CBHW041227270326
41934CB00001B/29